The New World of Cosmetic Treatments

How to Look Years Younger without Surgery

By Dr. Peter Ursel

Here's What's Inside...

Introduction

The New World of Cosmetic Treatments
June 2014
Ontario, Canada

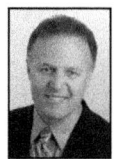 One of the things people often ask me is how they can avoid looking fake but still get all the benefits of using non-surgical cosmetic treatments. We've all seen the tabloids with the aging stars who have gone too far, and they look plastic and fake, or even in some cases like freaks.

I've been sharing how to look great without the risk of looking fake or plastic with my clients for years now with great success. In fact, inside this book I share with you my #1 cosmetic secret for looking younger but keeping you looking 100% like you. Your friends will wonder how you always look so refreshed and alive.

What follows is the transcript where I share with you the latest advance in cosmetic treatments, some of which will allow you to delay or even possibly forgo future cosmetic surgery altogether.

Enjoy the Book!

I hope this book educates you and helps change your way of thinking about your approach to beauty treatments and encourages you to take advantage of the new safer treatments that are available today.

Regards,

Dr. Peter Ursel

The New World of Cosmetic Treatments!

Ralph: Good afternoon, this is Ralph Trunfio and I'm here today with Dr. Peter Ursel from Ontario, Canada, who is going to share with us today his ideas about the new world of cosmetic treatments. Welcome Peter.

Peter: Thanks for having me.

Ralph: You've been practicing cosmetic treatment for some time now, many years as I recall. Is that correct?

Peter: Yes, I have been doing cosmetic treatment for almost 20 years now.

Ralph: Why do you want to write a book on beauty treatment?

Peter: I want to show people the new types of treatments that are available now that can make them look better without having a lot of downtime, discomfort or risk of looking "overdone." There is a lot of worry out there that getting cosmetic treatment or cosmetic surgery is going to be painful, or it's going to be something which causes them a lot of downtime.

Or they worry that it's going to make them look fake or too different from what they look like now to their friends. I'd like to reassure a lot of people with this book that that's no longer the case. There are new treatments available today which can make you look years and decades younger, but also retain a very natural look.

Why Does Our Face Age as We Get Older?

Ralph: That's exciting. I'm interested in hearing about these new treatments that are available. It seems like the face ages faster than any other part of our body. Why is that?

Peter: The whole body ages, but the face is a part of us that everyone sees and everyone focuses on when they look in the mirror. So it's not that the face ages faster than the rest of the body, it's that the face is our business card to the world if you will. So when we start to age, we tend to notice the changes in our face more so than other parts of our body.

To help people understand the facial aging process, I like to describe it by using the three Ds. The three Ds are deflation, descent and deterioration.

As you age you lose volume in the face. All the tissues lose volume, the bones shrink, the muscles shrink, and the skin shrinks. The fat underneath the skin shrinks. This is what we call Deflation. You get a deflation as the volume of all the tissues become less and less.

The second thing that happens as you age is you get a Descent. The skin is held up by the tissue underneath the skin, and with deflation things tend to fall down or descend.

Also, because the tissues don't have as much elastic tissue in them, they lose their elasticity, and they lose their spring. That is why tissue tends to descend or fall down because it doesn't have as much elasticity, and it doesn't spring back as much. That contributes to the descent as well as the loss of the volume. The volume is actually holding the skin up, and as you lose that volume the face tends to fall, and that changes the way we look.

The third thing that happens as we get older is the surface of the skin deteriorates. This is the third D, and there are lots of things that happen with that. The color of the skin changes; you develop brown spots and red spots and different sorts of lesions and moles and sometimes little skin cancers. You'll also notice the color of the skin changes, and the texture changes, but one of the big changes you'll see in the surface of the skin is it becomes more wrinkled with fine lines initially, and then as time goes on, as the volume decreases further, you get deeper folds and wrinkles in the skin.

The surface of the skin changes in that sense. The surface deteriorates; that's the third D. If you think of it in those three Ds, that gives you the three main reasons for the face to look like it's getting older.

The 3 Biggest Myths People Have regarding Cosmetic Beauty Treatments...

Ralph: Can you share with us some of the myths people have regarding cosmetic treatments?

Peter: One of the biggest myths people have is that cosmetic treatments are going to be painful, or there is going to be a large amount of discomfort. Fortunately due to improved technology, getting cosmetic treatments today is less painful than in the past. With modern anesthetic creams and better tools we use, most of the non-surgical cosmetic treatments are completely painless.

For example, cold air can be used to decrease the amount of discomfort which happens with certain treatments. We often use oral sedation which can help people relax before having some of the treatments.

The second myth or thing people worry about is looking significantly different from the way they look now. Most people want to look better but they don't want to look like somebody else. That's a big concern people have. I can assure them with the new technology we are going to talk about here that this does not have to be a concern.

The third myth is that you are going to be out of commission for an extended period of time from doing the treatments. They worry they won't look normal for months and months. This just isn't the case any longer. With modern beauty treatments, a lot of the downtime has been decreased significantly.

We are able to do the treatments with much less bruising and there is less chance of having scarring. Even redness has decreased with the newer treatment options available.

A final myth is that cosmetic beauty treatments are going to be really expensive. The truth is it can be relatively inexpensive or it can be very expensive depending on how much work people want. Usually we can customize treatments for people depending on their budget and the types of results they want.

Dr. Ursel's #1 Beauty Secret for Avoiding Looking Fake or Plastic...

Ralph: You mentioned earlier that people have a fear of looking fake or plastic. How can someone avoid this but still get the benefits that the treatments provide?

Peter: That's a big fear that people have of not looking like yourself. People want to look different, but they don't want anyone to notice that they've had surgery or treatments. You are walking a fine line there. You want to make them look better like they've been very refreshed without going too far and making them look like a different person.

You certainly see in the tabloids a lot now; you see pictures of some of the stars who have gone too far. People have huge lips or huge cheeks; their faces looking so tight that they're going to pop, or the skin looks super shiny, and that is a problem. There are some physicians that do that type of work, and some people insist on those treatments, but you don't have to do that. My approach to cosmetic treatments is to give people a very natural look. I really don't like the overdone look.

It's a big concern people have, and in fact I spend a lot of time reassuring them that that's not going to happen. When the treatments are done correctly, that is never a concern.

Ralph: You can help the patient look younger but still maintain a natural look?

Peter: Yes, in fact there are definitely ways of getting that natural look. One of the ways to get a natural look is to combine different types of treatments together. As I mentioned earlier there are three causes of aging: descent, deflation, and deterioration.

If you combine different treatments together and reverse those three things all at once, then you tend to get a really natural result, a synergistic result from combining different treatments together.

If you try to do everything with only one type of treatment, for example if you try to do everything with filler which helps with deflation, and you don't address the other two issues, descent and deterioration, then you can look a little bit plastic or overdone.

To avoid this, if you use a little bit less filler, and combine it with a skin treatment that smoothes the skin at the same time, then you can get a more natural appearance. Combining treatments together, rather than trying to do everything with a lot of one type of treatment, gives you a much more natural look.

Ralph: Very good. So the plastic look is created when someone only focuses on just one of the three areas?

Peter: Correct. In fact, the biggest secret I've learned in 20 years of cosmetic medicine is that you get the best results when you combine different classes of treatments together, and you do this consistently over time. Rather than pinning all your hopes on just one magic treatment, it is better to combine lesser amounts of different treatments, to get the natural result everyone craves.

How to Offset the Effects of Aging without Plastic Surgery...

Ralph: What are the treatments for each of the areas of the skin's three Ds?

Peter: Let's start with deflation. There are things that restore the volume underneath the skin. For example fillers such as Restylane and Juvederm and other different brands of fillers on the market add and restore the volume underneath the skin.

There are also treatments which restore the volume right in the skin surface itself. I'm excited about this new option. There are now fillers you can use right in the skin's surface itself to restore the volume within the skin cells. This is a new treatment which has just come over from Europe to North America. This new treatment is especially helpful for restoring the thin skin of the neck and around the eyes which until now have been very difficult to improve.

You can also inject fat underneath the skin to restore volume. Those are the things that can address deflation. When you address deflation, you are lifting up the skin.

How to Combat Descent...

Adding volume helps to lift up things to reverse descent, but you can also do things that will tighten up the skin. For example, there are several new devices that are available that use radio frequency energy. They use a type of heat to tighten up the skin and tighten up the collagen within the skin.

Another option for battling the descent of the skin is to use other sources of energy like ultrasound. This special ultrasound device uses focused ultrasound beams to tighten up the skin.

Of course there is always the extreme example of tightening by doing surgery where you actually cut the skin out, and that tightens things right up. That would be the extreme method of addressing descent, but for our purposes we are not really talking about surgical treatments. In fact, with the new treatments that are available, surgical options can be pushed further and further down the path.

How to Address the Deterioration of the Surface of the Skin...

Ralph: That's exciting that the new treatments are improving so much. What about deterioration? This is an area that a lot of people struggle with. What are the options for the deterioration of the skin on the face?

Peter: To address deterioration of the surface of the skin is, in fact, where most of the modern treatments are used. There are different lasers which can actually take off the surface levels of the skin in various depths, and there are special lasers that can actually make little holes in the skin that stimulate the collagen to be reformed, and that can be used especially for scarring of the skin.

There are special types of lasers that will actually just remove pigmentation from the skin which are called intense pulse light or broadband light treatments. These can be used to address the pigmentation changes in the skin. There are also treatments like microdermabrasion and chemical peels, and those can be used to take off a small layer of the skin.

Additionally, you can use the various different types of creams and lotions. There are a lot of good creams that can actually have an anti-aging effect on the skin's surface. Generally speaking those are the ways that you can address the deterioration of the skin's surface.

When you look at all the different categories of treatments, and you combine them together in a skillful way, you can get a really natural restoration of your look.

Why Botox Is Not the Filler You Think It Is...

Ralph: In these treatments for the different types of deterioration, where does Botox fall?

Peter: That's a good question because many people get that mixed up. They look at Botox as sort of being a generic treatment that treats everything. Actually Botox is a treatment that goes underneath the skin and into the muscle. When Botox is injected into a muscle, it causes that muscle to relax. It's used specifically in places where lines on the surface of the skin are caused by excessive muscle action or repetitive muscle action, for example in the frown area.

A lot of people have frown lines between their eyes; that's the most common place that Botox is used. It can also be used on the crow's feet area where you see little lines forming from repetitive smiling. When you relax those muscles in that area, you tend to get an improvement in the lines in that area. You can use it on the forehead to address the forehead lines, but you must be careful you don't use too much because you can make the whole area look inactive because it relaxes the muscles and it can make you look stiff. You've got to be very careful with that.

The other thing that can happen with too much Botox is the brow can drop a little bit. Botox works purely by relaxing the muscles and the main area to use it is in the area around the eyes. Botox is mainly used in the upper half of the face, though it is increasingly being used in other areas as well.

Ralph: So Botox is not a filler as I erroneously thought it was.

Peter: A lot of people think Botox is the same as filler, whereas the filler works just by adding volume underneath and pumping up a wrinkle or a line. Fillers can also be used to bring up the cheeks or lift the face. You can do almost a full face lift now with fillers, but they act by adding volume and lifting. The fillers are completely different from Botox.

Ralph: How long am I going to be laid up with a Botox treatment? Is there a typical amount of recovery time for that?

Peter: There is no downtime whatsoever with Botox. In fact you don't get bruising from using Botox. The thing with Botox is it usually takes about three days to work to fully see the results.

How New Technology Has Revolutionized Fillers...

Ralph: What about fillers?

Peter: With fillers there can be downtime because sometimes you can get a bit of swelling or bruising from the treatment. However with newer techniques of using fillers where we use special blunt needles called cannulas, there is much less bruising now than there used to be. Just in the last year and a half, I have incorporated the use of cannulas into my practice, and you see much less bruising now because they really don't cut the blood vessels. When they go under the skin, they gently deposit the filler where you want it to go.

Only about 5-10% of physicians are using the cannulas to deliver fillers now. It's a new technique. The way you use them is you use a tiny hollow needle with a blunt tip on the end. Most needles have a sharp tip on them. The cannulas look like a needle but if you look at them closely, the tip of them is blunt. You can actually push it in your finger, and it wouldn't cut you. There is a little side port in the cannula where the filler comes out.

That's really different from the traditional method of injecting filler where there is a sharp needle that goes underneath the skin. When you are at the skin's surface, you can see where the needle is. You can see it pierce the skin, but when you are underneath the skin, you can't see what's happening, and there are all kinds of blood vessels under the skin that if you hit them with a needle, you can bleed, and you can get a lot of bruising as a result.

That's what traditionally causes the bruising, whereas with the cannula you make a little hole in the skin that you can see, and then you gently put the cannula into that hole. Then you push the little blood vessels to the side, so that you don't get any bruising whatsoever with them.

The cannulas have really revolutionized where you can put the fillers because there are some places on the face where there are blood vessels that you really have to be careful of. However now with the cannula, you can be sure you are not going to pierce a blood vessel or accidentally inject some of the material into a blood vessel. It really made a huge difference for the safety and success of these treatments.

Ralph: Because a lot of the downtime you see is recovering from the bruises from the old method of using a needle to inject the filler?

Peter: Exactly. We almost never see any bruising with the fillers going in, and that used to be very unpredictable. If you hit a blood vessel, you could have a big bruise that can be there for a full week, whereas now I can be just about 99% sure that there is going to be no bruising whatsoever.

Because there's been a big improvement in technology in this area, there is much less downtime. I used to tell people with fillers that they could have swelling and lumpiness and bumps and things like that for a few days up to five days. Now with the new techniques, they can literally come in and go to a party that evening with no down time and instantly look better. Sometimes there is an exception if you do your lips. Sometimes lips can be a little bit swollen, but there is really not much downtime at all with any of the filler treatments.

Ralph: When you say downtime, can you define that for us? What do you mean by downtime?

Peter: There is the social downtime where you don't want to be seen by other people, but it doesn't mean that you are incapacitated, that you can't go out. It's just you may need to use some make up. Whereas medical downtime is where your face can be swollen, and you can look a little bit disfigured for a time.

That's what we are trying to stay away from here, but most of the time downtime is just the amount of time where it looks like you had treatment done; people can see that you have had something done. We are trying to minimize that, so that you don't have to miss any work at all and are able to return to your activities right away after the treatment.

Why Skin Tighteners Will Give You a Great Lifting Effect...

Ralph: Let's talk about the skin tighteners now. How do those work?

Peter: Skin tighteners work by using different types of heat. The most common one is radio frequency which is a type of energy. When these skin tightening units are put on the skin, they heat up the collagen in the skin.

If you imagine the collagen to be like little springs in the skin that hold the skin up and keep it tight, what happens over time is these little springs unravel and become lax. When you pick up the skin, it just doesn't snap back the way it used to because the collagen has done two things: First of all there is less collagen; secondly it's become kind of loose. When you heat the collagen up, it tightens up like a spring, and it makes the skin tighter which gives it a lifting effect.

You can't really get a huge amount of lifting with this, but you can get some lifting and some tightening up of the skin in people between the ages of let's say 35 and 55, and that can be a significant improvement. As you get beyond 55 to 60, there is less and less collagen in the skin, so the skin tighteners don't tend to work as well. The other thing is there tends to be a lot more loosening at that point. You can get results, but they just wouldn't be as good as someone who is younger.

There are newer skin tighteners available now. One in particular is very exciting. It uses ultrasound energy, and it uses a fair amount of ultrasound energy to heat up the tissue underneath the skin and give you even more skin tightening. It's a little bit more painful and a quite a bit more expensive, but it's a newer technology that can be used to tighten up the skin to give a fresh healthy look.

Ralph: How long do skin tightening treatments typically last?

Peter: There are different types of skin tightening treatments on the market. There are those where you go for a one time treatment, and then there are those where you go for a series of treatments. The ones where there is a series of treatments, there is no discomfort, and there is a gradual tightening over the space of six weeks. You may want to do six treatments for example. You could expect those results to last probably a year, and then you may want to repeat it one or two treatments every year to maintain your results.

You can get results which last six months to a year with the skin tightener, but it also depends on other things that you are doing because we usually combine the skin tighteners with fillers and other treatment modalities. It is difficult to say exactly when one treatment wears out. What we suggest to people if they are going to do skin tightening is to do it yearly for maintenance.

Ralph: That is longer than I would have thought. Since we are heating up the collagen, why when it cools down does this not reverse the effect?

Peter: What happens is when you heat up the skin like that, you tend to get an initial tightening up and then a little bit of a loosening. That is what happens with our particular machine. You can actually see the skin tightening up in front of you, you can see an improvement right away, and then it loosens a bit. Then that effect will sort of gradually reverse itself, and then if you repeat it within a week, you get it before it reverses completely.

When you stack the treatments on top of each other, you tend to get a more permanent type of tightening with the skin, rather than just that initial short term effect. An extreme example is someone who has had a burn. When you have a burn on your skin, part of the problem is that you get extreme contractures and a lot of the physical therapy that people have afterward is to loosen up the contracture because there is so much collagen in burnt skin. An extreme burn will give you an extreme tightening, but you obviously can't see that when you are doing a cosmetic treatment. That's what we are trying to do. You are trying to get enough heating to cause tightening of the skin without burning the skin.

Ralph: Is there much downtime with these?

Peter: Generally speaking there is no downtime at all with the skin tightening treatments; that's what's nice about them. You can come in and have them, and there is no downtime.

How to Avoid Downtime and Get the Results You Want...

Ralph: As a rule how much downtime from the laser treatments?

Peter: It just depends completely on how much or how deep of a treatment you do. A surface laser treatment can give you absolutely no downtime; it just looks like you have a little bit of a sunburn, whereas a deep laser peel can give you up to a week of downtime or even more than that, especially if you remove a lot of the skin surface.

But there is less downtime than there used to be with a lot of these treatments because the technologies have improved so much. With the laser that I have, you can go anywhere from 4 microns to

200 microns. To put things in perspective a microdermabrasion treatment that you typically get will remove about two microns in depth. The lowest level our laser will go is about four microns, which is about twice as much as a microdermabrasion.

That gives you a little bit of sunburn. If you have a 200 micro laser peel, then the skin is going to be raw and possibly oozing a little bit. That's the extreme depth of that type of treatment. If you do four passes or three passes of 200 microns, you are getting 600 microns. You can imagine if you go to that kind of depth in the skin, it's going be very raw and will need to heal over the space of about a week to 10 days. The effect however, will be very noticeable, once the skin heals.

To recap, you can go anywhere from a little burn type of effect right up to having your skin oozing and being swollen for a week. That's all controllable though, with the technology we have now we can control exactly how many microns someone wants to go deep with our people and the energy we want to use.

Ralph: Whether or not you go deeper depends on what outcome you are trying to achieve?

Peter: Yes, for example if you look at people that have deep lines around their lips and around their mouths, those are deep lines and you can improve them with a little bit of filler underneath the skin. However to get the really good results with that, you need to actually peel the surface of the skin to compensate for as deep as those lines are. Some of those lines can be as deep as 800 microns.

You might have to go quite deep to reverse that. If you have the deep lines around your mouth and you want to have them removed, you are going to have to expect some downtime to get the results you want. Generally speaking, though, most of the treatments except for the deep surfacing treatments don't have much down time.

How to Get the Synergistic Advantage of Doing Multiple Treatments at Once...

Ralph: Very good. So someone can choose to have the deeper treatments or not. Let's talk a bit more about the advantages of combining the different treatments.

Peter: When you combine different types of treatments, you are actually treating the cause of the aging face. When you combine different classes of treatments, you actually treat more of the causes of aging. The more of the causes you address, the more that you are going to reverse all those causes.

If you just reverse one of the causes of aging, for example if you just add volume and don't address the skin issue, then you are just treating one aspect of what causes you to look aged. What happens when you do this is it doesn't look right. It won't look as good as when you combine the different treatments together. When you combine treatments you get not just an added effect you get a synergistic effect like adding 1+1 to equal 3 instead of 2.

The different treatments act synergistically when you address more than one of the causes of aging.

How Advancement in Technology Has Reduced the Need for Surgical Solutions...

Ralph: Are you suggesting that today with the improvements in the technology of beauty treatments, you can avoid going under the knife?

Peter: What you can do is you can delay going under the knife. There are several reasons to try to delay or avoid plastic surgery. First of all plastic surgery tends to be more expensive than what we are discussing today.

The second thing is there tends to be more risks with surgery because you have to have a general anesthetic, and there's cutting involved, and that has a higher risk for infection and for complications.

Third thing is that surgery is more drastic, so the risk of looking significantly different is bigger, which as we discussed, is a big concern for a lot of people.

Having said that, there are a lot of problems that non-surgical cosmetic treatments simply will not address. For example if you've got really loose eyelids, laser treatments are very difficult to improve these. Sometimes you need to have the surgery to cut out some of the loose skin. If you have a lot of extra skin around your neck, surgery is going to be the best thing for you. You may not want to have surgery because it's too expensive, or your problem can be solved with non-surgical methods, but sometimes surgery has its place and is necessary to get the results that you want.

It just depends on the type of problem you are dealing with, your budget and your tolerance for downtime.

Ralph: If someone uses the cosmetic treatments you've discussed with us today, can they put off the need for surgery for years?

Peter: That's right; you can put off the need for surgery. You can have treatments that are less expensive and with zero down time. The other thing is by putting things off, you are also giving technology a chance to re-develop and surgery may possibly be put off forever. By doing the treatments available today, you are buying yourself time because the technology every year changes and improves.

For example in the space of five years, laser technology has improved dramatically. If you can put off surgery for five years with this pace and change in technology, you can see things happen which in the future are going to make a lot of the cosmetic surgeries unnecessary. It's quite exciting actually.

Ralph: Yeah, it is exciting. Can you speak to the fear someone may have that once they start these treatments, they won't be able to stop using them?

Peter: There are no treatments that I'm aware of where things actually get worse after the treatment has stopped. For example if you do Botox and you stop doing it, you are not going to look worse than you did before you did the Botox. In fact in some of these treatments, you will have a very long positive residual effect.

The other thing is once you start to get the good results and you see good results, you will want to have more of them. That's very common. Success with beauty treatments is very impactful.

You can become excited by the new things that are happening. One of the doctors' jobs is to be careful. There are people that tend to want more done. One of my jobs is to say no to people at times; it's to say, "No, you don't need more filler. You don't need more laser treatments." That is part of the art of this. It is to be judicious and selective in the treatments that you use.

Ralph: We come in and have a treatment and like the result, so we think having more treatments done would equal more success.

Peter: One of the things is you see that a little bit of filler is good, the lips look good, and then the next thing you know the lips are bigger, and before you know it the lips are big, and you look somewhat ridiculous.

Ralph: Sometimes less is more. Can you share with us what the results of using these treatments are? Is there a way to quantify this?

Peter: We have a lot of people who look five to ten years younger, and you can reverse a lot of those changes we discussed as we age. We haven't achieved a state where we can stop aging completely, but we can reverse a lot of the changes we see. Then with maintenance treatment, we can maintain those results over time. Looking five to ten years younger is not unreasonable. Everyone is different. Some people have super deep wrinkles which can be genetic.

I can see two ladies, both aged 55, and one will be completely wrinkled, and the other one will have beautiful skin depending on genetics and how well she has taken care of herself over the years. The skin tends to show a lot of lifestyle and history on the skin. You can tell by looking at someone how much they've been outside, their genetics, and how well they take care of themselves.

There are a lot of factors involved that are beyond what I do, but we can make people look five to ten years younger.

Ralph: We talked about the 3 Ds and the treatments of the 3 Ds as though they were different problems, different solutions. I imagine you have patients who get a myriad of treatments, not just a treatment for a single defect, but multiple treatments for whatever is ailing them at the time. Is that true?

Peter: That's true. To get the best results as I mentioned earlier, most people should have combinations of treatments. I like to think of it in three phases. In the first phase I like to get a really rapid and dramatic initial result for somebody. Using fillers and using some laser resurfacing will usually get people a fast initial change, and then after that you are going to do treatments that are going to give you a more gradual improvement.

In the second phase we see slower results that build on the first phase treatments. For example skin tightening is something that is spaced over six weeks and works more gradually. Another treatment that can take more time to see results is the new skin filler that actually works in the skin surface over a period 3 months with treatments being done every 30 days. In the third phase, you use maintenance treatments, where you use skin creams and periodic repeats of the treatments we've talked about earlier, to maintain and continue to improve over the months and the years that follow.

In summary those initial treatments give you a fairly fast positive result, and then we follow up with slower ones soon after. Then for long term maintenance we like to use skin care products and periodic repeats with some of the other treatments such as Botox, fillers and laser treatments.

Here Are the Answers to Commonly Asked Cosmetic Treatment Questions...

Ralph: What can you tell us, Peter, about the systemic treatments, things the patient can do on their own where they don't have to be in your office?

Peter: That's a huge area, the whole area of anti-aging medicine. For example hormonal treatments can have an effect on aging as can nutritional products, and some vitamins. Our skin care products tend to have vitamins in them. We like to have a more nutritional approach for the skin and not use harsh chemicals on the skin.

Those can also be augmented by taking supplements as well and by eating a good diet. A more natural diet that's high in vegetables is going to cause your skin to look better. The other thing, too, is protecting your skin against the sun. Sunscreens, using hats, and things like that – limiting your sun exposure – that can help.

For example if you smoke cigarettes and you quit smoking, your skin is going to look a lot better. What happens when you smoke cigarettes is you get constriction of blood vessels, and you don't get as much blood going to the surface of the skin. Typically someone who quits smoking will have an improvement in the color and tone of their skin.

Those are systemic things you can do or types of lifestyle changes you can make. Definitely improving your diet, quitting smoking, protecting your skin from sun exposure and exercising will improve your skin. Exercising has a beneficial effect because you get more blood flow to the skin surface, which improves the skin.

Ralph: What can you tell us about skin care products?

Peter: What I can say is that I didn't use to believe this, but if someone uses the right type of skin care products in conjunction with what we do at the office that's probably going to be 30% of the results that they get. You are not only going to get improvements, but you are going to maintain any of the results that we get in the office with our laser treatments and other different types of skin surface treatments.

The most important thing that you should probably have in your skin care products is sunblock. You should also have vitamin A and vitamin C. Those are the three main ingredients that skin care products should have in them. The vitamin A actually helps to stabilize the skin cells and returns them to a normal state. If it's in the right sort of mixture, vitamin C can have an anti-oxidant type of effect.

It protects the skin from free radicals which are caused by things like cigarette smoke, toxins in the environment, and the sun. All those things contribute to free radical formation which causes aging and changes the pigmentation and the color of the skin. Using vitamin C helps to reverse that and protects the skin. Vitamin A, vitamin C, and a good sun block are really essential for people if they are going to continue to get improvements and protect their skin.

Ralph: What can you tell us about helping with the appearance of our neck?

Peter: The neck is an area that is getting more and more attention now because so many people are getting great results on their facial skin. Their face will look great, but then their neck will...there will be a disconnect. The neck will look 10 years, 15 years older than their face. Part of the reason for that is the emphasis is on the face, but now there's more attention given to the neck and the top of the chest area.

We are now extending our treatments down to that area and suggesting that people use their skin care products on their necks and chest as well. One of the other problems is that the skin on the neck is very thin, and it's been difficult to treat the neck with lasers because you really can't go too deep with the lasers. Now with the new lasers you can control the depth much more precisely, and you can treat the neck skin very safely.

The other thing with the neck is you can also treat the pigmentation with different products and BBL (Broad Band Light) treatments. Another big development in the last year or so is new products mostly from Europe that actually are like fillers but they don't add volume underneath the skin.

They get injected right into the skin surface, and they rehydrate the skin. You see, one of the ingredients that is now commonly in skin care products is called hyaluronic acid. Hyaluronic acid is something that is in the skin cells. When it decreases, the skin cells tend to deflate and lose their shiny appearance.

There have been all kinds of efforts to put hyaluronic acid into creams, but it really doesn't get absorbed well. There are products that can be injected into the skin that go in directly. They bypass the skin's surface and go directly into the skin cells. By plumping up the little skin cells in the neck, you can get a huge improvement in the thickness of the skin and make the skin more dense in the neck.

That has been a major new event in the last year or so, and it's come from Europe. There is lots of hope now for people's necks because as well as using laser treatment and skin care products we can now use these new special fillers to improve the way the neck looks.

Ralph: What if a person has generally thin skin? Is there anything they can do to fix or improve upon that?

Peter: That is the million dollar question. There are treatments which can stimulate the skin, that thicken up the skin. They are designed to help the collagen, and that's what some of the skin tighteners are supposed to do, to thicken up the skin. There's not much available on the market now except these new fillers. That's where I'm seeing a lot of these improvements now with these new special injectable products that can actually thicken the skin. They make the skin cells thicker.

To restore collagen to the skin and to add collagen is difficult, but the products will help. Some of the topical products like Vitamin C can actually help restore collagen in the skin. The problem is absorption of these products, and that's one of the major areas of research at the moment, increasing the thickness of the skin.

Ralph: Let's hope they continue to come up with fantastic new ways to help people in this area. Are there specific treatments that address Rosacea, or redness of the face?

Peter: Yes. There are some really good laser treatments available now, such as laser light devices that can treat Rosacea. They go by the name of Broadband Light or Intense Post Light or the short forms are BBL and IPL. These are special lights that, when the light hits the redness on the skin, those areas absorb more energy. What happens is that energy causes the little blood vessels to close down which is what is causing the redness on the surface of the skin.

These types of laser instruments in combination with the right type of cream can really improve overall redness in the skin. Some people's skin needs medical treatment as well. For example if you have acne or Rosacea, antibiotics are useful; there are special creams which can be used. There are special prescription creams which can be used to help to minimize the redness.

The most dramatic results for the redness of the skin is achieved with the laser Broad Band Light or as we call it BBL.

Ralph: What can you tell us about the process for getting rid of moles?

Peter: That's another huge area. The first part of the solution for moles is to actually have a physician look at the mole to diagnose it. Depending on the type of mole, skin bump, or lesion on the skin, the treatment is customized. The most important thing is to make sure the mole in question is not a cancerous growth.

That's why it's important to have it looked at by a physician initially, and once the type of mole has been determined, then there are several different ways to remove them. There are surgical treatments that can be used where the mole is actually cut out, and plastic surgery stitches are used to repair the little defect.

Liquid nitrogen is a very cold treatment and can be used on raised lesions. We can also use lasers to treat some types of moles. Another method used to treat a flat pigmented area is the intense pulse light or broad band light (BBL) treatment. As you can see there are several different types of treatments available for moles but the most important part is getting a good diagnosis at the beginning, and then a plan can be made from there depending on the diagnosis.

Ralph: Are there lifestyles that can lead to skin cancer?

Peter: The most important thing is to avoid, or at the very least minimize, exposure to the sun. We see a lot of skin cancers on the face, the ears and the areas that have been exposed to the sun over the years. Certainly smoking and drinking alcohol will make you more predisposed to skin cancer. A family history of skin cancer also makes you more prone to skin cancer.

Some skin types are also more prone to skin cancer, for example very light skin or fair hair. Red heads are more prone to developing skin cancer. The reason is they have less melanin in their skin which protects them from sun exposure.

Ralph: How are these treatments different from what I would get if I was just going to a spa? Is there a distinction about what you are talking about and what you can get when you go to the same place that you get your nails done?

Peter: A lot of the spas are now offering more of these treatments, however there is less regulation at spas, and some of the technology that's used in the spas tends to be less expensive or not as good. The patient is taking a bit more of a risk when they go to a beauty spa for cosmetic treatments.

The staff is not medically educated either. They don't have the knowledge of the structure of the skin and all the skin diseases to look out for. One of the big things we look for is skin cancer. My nurse and my staff are always looking for different tell-tale signs of skin cancer. We pick up a lot of skin cancer in people where they didn't think they had it. I hate to think what would happen if they just went to their local spa and hadn't come into our office for treatments.

I think you are better off going to a facility where there are medically trained people to get your skin treatments. Also, sometimes people need prescription medications which can only be provided by a physician, and they are not available at a spa.

There are prescription treatments for different types of skin disorders like acne and Rosacea, different types of skin cancer, even different creams to treat skin cancer. We can do more advanced treatments with our clients because we can use anesthetics as well as use special topical anesthetics and oral medication which you can't get from a spa.

Here's Exactly How You Can Look Years Younger without Surgery…

Ralph: We've covered a lot of ground here. How can I find out what's the best combination of treatments for me?

Peter: The most important thing to do if you are interested in having cosmetic treatments is to try and educate yourself, and that's what this book is for: to understand the different types of beauty treatments that are available. The second thing if you want to go further is to come in and have a special consultation with the physician to go over the different types of problems that you have. An evaluation can be made for the 3 Ds for your face, and then a plan can be put together.

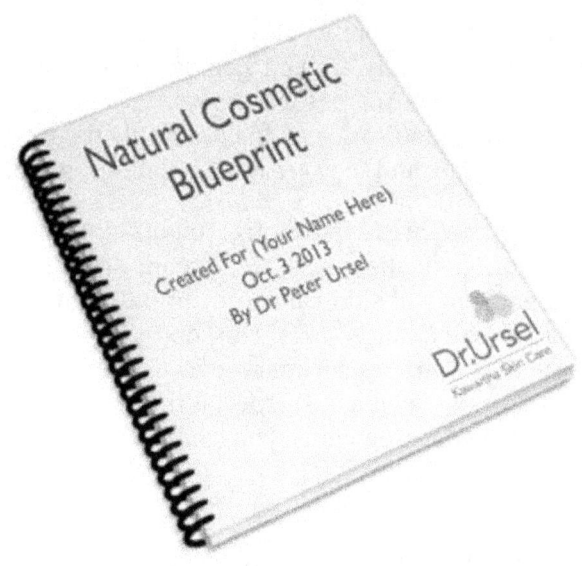

We have something called a Natural Cosmetic Blueprint, an actual cosmetic blue print that we create for people when they come in to see us. We do a full skin consultation and go over all of the issues and concerns you have, and then depending on what we find, what your goals are, and what your budget is, we put together a blueprint that we follow over the next several months to give you the results that you want.

Ralph: Is this something I can walk out of your office with, or are they are delivered to me after the consultation?

Peter: Once we've had the consultation we put the blueprint on paper and then that can be emailed or it can be mailed. We put it on a chart that we use as a guide for our treatment. It is not carved in stone because there is some flexibility in this, but it is nice to have a plan set out for you when you decide you want to do it.

Ralph: I'm hoping it will identify a plan that if I were the patient I would have ways of recalling what the bigger plan is, so it can refresh my memory after the fact.

Peter: That's right. That's what the blueprint does. We come up with a plan, and we put things on a calendar and go from there.

Ralph: If the reader has an interest in getting their own blueprint how should they contact you to go to the next step?

Peter: The best thing to do is to call our office at 705-328-1747 and tell them that you would like to be assessed properly and have a natural cosmetic blue print put together, and we can arrange that. You can also go to my website to get more information on the different treatments at www.doctorursel.com.

Ralph: Very interesting conversation, very informative. Thank you very much for giving us your time and sharing this information with us.

Peter: My pleasure. It's my passion to help people have beautiful, natural looking skin. The most important thing to remember always is that you will get the best and most natural results with the skillful and careful combination of the 3 different categories of treatments. With consistent treatments done regularly over time, there is a compounding effect of the different treatments. I find this makes a profound difference in the results that we achieve.

Here's How to Look Years Younger without Surgery...

You already know that taking care of your skin is an important part of looking good. The confusing part is not knowing the new beauty treatments available to look years younger without looking fake or unnatural.

That's where we come in. We help people just like you look 10 year younger without surgery.

Step 1: We invest 45 minutes with you doing a special consultation and evaluation on your skin and problem areas.

Step 2: We design your customized Natural Cosmetic Blueprint based on the results of the consultation and the goals you desire.

Step 3: We take it from here and implement the blueprint to get your skin looking fresh and healthy.

Most people think it takes suffering through painful cosmetic treatments with lots of downtime to look great.

Now you can look years younger with no or very little downtime and with minimal pain.

If you'd like us to help, just call 705 328 1747 or send an email to: kawarthasc@gmail.com and we will take it from there.

About the Author

Dr. Peter Ursel lives in the city of Kawartha Lakes and has been doing cosmetic and leg vein treatments for over 20 years. He initially worked as a family physician and then did emergency medicine full time for 10 years. During this time he developed the skills necessary to do all the procedures that he currently performs full time at his clinic in Lindsay Ontario.

Testimonials

"I would recommend Dr. Ursel to any of my friends. He explains any procedure in depth. Everyone is pleasant and very professional."

S.L.

******

"My initial visit when I met the friendly staff, I received a complimentary dermabrasion and had Dr. Ursel explain what treatments could improve the condition of my skin by removing age spots, evening skin tone, smoothing texture, and even reducing wrinkles; in fact, providing a more youthful appearance. I have always received courteous, friendly professional service and have been very pleased with the improvement to my skin as a result of a combination of laser treatments, chemical peels and dermabrasion. I also appreciate being able to buy excellent products to complement the treatments."

F.F.

******

"The staff was friendly and made me feel at ease. The doctor and nurse were very professional, but at the same time, very caring and considerate. I recommend laser treatments, if possible; it is not a painful procedure, and you can continue your normal activities - within reason."

E.S.

******

"I had estelux (laser like treatment) on my face because it was very red, and I also had spider veins on my face. The results are amazing. I love my face, have a lot of confidence, and I feel like a new woman. The staff is great, makes me feel great just walking in to the office. It was an experience I can't forget. I will continue coming now for my other imperfections because I believe in Dr. Ursel and trust his judgment."

M.G.

******

"Having suffered from Rosacea for over fifteen years, I had given up finding a cure that really works. When I became aware of your treatment, (Estelux), I admit I was skeptical of the whole idea. However with the help of my husband, I pushed myself to visit you. Best decision of my life. Much to my surprise I cannot express enough how grateful I am to you.

Discomfort was minimal and did not interfere with my daily life. The result was more than I ever hoped for. Now, when I look in the mirror, I love what I see. A confident, new woman!"

M.G.

******

"Facial laser treatment for moles, sun damage, age spots. My husband and I really appreciated the complimentary skin examination to detect early signs of skin cancer."

******